# Food

# and

# Me

# and

# the Bible

The truths in the Bible changed my relationship with food.

By Judith A. Eastham

Copyright © 2019 Judith A. Eastham

All rights reserved.

ISBN 979-8-6406-5402-8

No part of this publication may be reproduced, distributed, or transmitted in any form or by any means, including photocopying, recording, or other electronic or mechanical methods, or by any information storage and retrieval system without the prior written permission of the publisher, except in the case of very brief quotations embodied in critical reviews and certain other noncommercial uses permitted by copyright law.

All scriptures used are King James, taken from the KING JAMES VERSION (KJV): KING JAMES VERSION, public domain.

# Table of contents

82

# Appreciations

I have wanted to write this story for a long time.  God gave me a desire to share what I had learned so I could help and encourage others.  My goal is that this book will help you let God and his word, the Bible, lead you to better health.

I want to give appreciation to Sophia Tucker of Tapestry of Beauty Ministries and author of *Renewing the Mind 101*.  I had already begun writing when she said, "Judith, why don't you write a book?"  It was the push I needed to get moving on it.

I also want to thank all who helped me in this journey of reducing my weight and making improvements in my health.  There are too many to mention, but when I found the Thin Within program, I was able to begin making permanent changes.  Their books, classes, and workbooks were beneficial.  They led me to Barb Raveling's books.  She uses the word of God and leads a person to apply it to their physical health.

I also want to thank Beth Callaghan of the Tapestry of Beauty Ministries with the editing and encouragement she gave.

# Preface

"Good grief! Who is snoring? It woke me up," this was thought in my mind as I groggily woke up.  It was still the middle of the night. "Oh, no," I groaned.  "It was me. My own snoring woke me up!"  My husband was working the night shift, and I was the only one in bed.

I lay there thinking after I turned my achy body in bed. "It's even hard to turn.  I am at the highest weight of my life.  I don't know what to do."  When I woke up, my head bending back to let my windpipe open up caused my neck to ache.   My joints ached because my joints always seemed to hurt when I had too much sugar.

I was so miserable.  I could not remember being so physically miserable before.  It made me sad.  I was worried because I felt so hopeless.  I would start a diet, but sometimes I couldn't last more than three days.  Sure, I had lost weight before.  I knew how.  I had a shelf full of diet books.  Plus, I had read a lot of books on nutrition. Food and nutrition had always been a favorite topic of mine.  It was not a lack of education.  I was a nurse and had a college-level science class in nutrition.

What was the problem?  I began to pray, "Oh, God, I am in a terrible mess.  You have helped me before.  You showed me the way, and I have gone away from what you showed me.  I need help."

I wish I could say I made a permanent change that day. I did not. It was many "diets" later. It took a life jarring illness and death of a diet buddy and sister at church to make me take notice enough to make a permanent change.

In this book are some of what I learned as I applied God's truth to this part of my life. If you are feeling hopeless, I hope sharing my experience will help you. Each chapter ends with some questions to think about, pray about, and journal. Get a Bible, a journal, and be ready to change.

# CHAPTER 1 - IN THE BEGINNING

Food, and me.  I and food have had a stormy relationship, which is weird since food is an inanimate object.  Why would I even have a relationship with food at all? I also have a long relationship with the God of the Bible.  I believe the Bible is the Word of God and is infallible, without error, and a guide for my life.

Let's go back to the beginning.  No, not my beginning relationship with food.  The beginning of the Bible.  In the beginning, God made it all, including all the plants and animals and people and said it was good.  In fact, he says human creation was very good.  It had God's approval.

The first relationship between humans and the food was this.  God said in Genesis 2:9 "And out of the ground made the LORD God to grow every tree that is pleasant to the sight, and good for food; the tree of life also in the midst of the garden, and the tree of knowledge of good and evil."  In Genesis 2: 16 and 17 he said, "And the LORD God commanded the man, saying, 'Of every tree of the garden thou mayest freely eat: But of the tree of the knowledge of good and evil, thou shalt not eat of it: for in the day that thou eatest thereof thou shalt surely die.'"

So that was what God had to say about people and their relationship with food.  He made humans need food for physical nourishment.  They had the natural mechanism for hunger so they would grow and stay healthy.  And, he supplied what they needed.  He told them to eat freely.  He did give them a boundary.  He also gave them a consequence for breaking the boundary.

And they all lived happily ever after.

Sigh, no, we wish.  No, that was not how it went.  The first humans questioned the boundary.  Why would the boundary be disputed?  God gave humans free will.  He wanted them to obey him, but he wanted them to follow him of their own free will.  He had also made many animals who had a natural hunger, and they ate whatever they wanted.  They ate entirely by instinct.  He wanted some creature that had a choice to love him.  He wanted them to obey Him out of love and not because they had to.  He was their creator and loved them like they were his children.  He visited them every evening in the Garden of Eden and had a loving relationship with them.

So, this is what happened. The story is in Genesis, chapter 3.  The serpent, who was possessed by Satan, came and talked to Eve in the garden.  It may have gone like this. The serpent said to Eve, "Hasn't God said you could eat of every tree in the garden?"

Eve replied, "Yes, he has, all except one. He said we could not eat of the tree of knowledge of good and evil. We are not even to touch it, or we will die." Now God had not said they couldn't touch it, but she added to it.

Satan replied, "You won't really die. Let me tell you the real story. If you eat of it, God knows you will be like gods, and you will know about both good and evil."

This information got Eve thinking. She thought, "Well, if I won't die, maybe the consequences aren't so bad." So, she took a closer look at the fruit. It looked good to eat. It was a beautiful fruit. "It does look like it is from a tree that will make me wise. I want to be wise. I won't have to study so hard with Adam, learning all the names he has given the plants and animals. I will be wise and already know! In fact, I think he could use a little wisdom too. I will eat some and also offer some to him."

So, she did. Adam was so charmed by her explanation; he ate of the fruit of the tree. He may have thought, "This woman God has given me, I knew she was beautiful, but I think she is also brilliant! I think she is right! I will eat some too and gain more wisdom! It will make it so easy to know everything." Or it might have been quite a bit simpler than that. Adam may have thought, "Well, it looks good, and she seems okay. Why not try it? Maybe I will be more like God. I would like that."

Oh, the reasoning of us humans. If we want something, we can always find a way to make it sound like the very best thing to do.

The consequences of their actions were anything but good.  What they did learn was the difference between good and evil.  Obeying God was doing good and disobeying God was doing evil.  It was that simple.  They also learned about the consequences of disobeying God.  It was far worse than they ever thought it would be.  They learned about the death God said were the consequences.  It was spiritual death.  It was a death that separated them from God.

Physically they were now separated from God.  God moved them out of his garden.  He never let them return.

It was also spiritual death.  He did continue to be their God, but the relationship was changed.  He still loved them as a father loves his children, but they had to confess and repent of their sin.  Repentance restored the relationship but did not remove the consequences.  Their respect for God and his sovereignty increased.

Journal questions:

1.  What lessons about boundaries do you see in this story?
2.  What are your thoughts about the limits God sets as boundaries?
3.  In your life, are boundaries lines rules to break, or are they guidelines to protect you?
4.  What are your thoughts about the possibility that God would give you boundaries with your eating or drinking?

# CHAPTER 2 - WHY BOUNDARIES?

Why would God give boundaries?  We saw in the last chapter that God wanted someone to obey him because they loved him.  He loved them.  He had made them and wanted to fellowship with them.

So why would boundaries be needed?  Couldn't we live happily without limits, doing what we wanted and when we wanted?  Let us look at some scripture.

Jeremiah 31:1, 3 "At the same time, saith the LORD, will I be the God of all the families of Israel, and they shall be my people.  The LORD hath appeared of old unto me, saying, Yea, I have loved thee with an everlasting love: therefore with lovingkindness have I drawn thee."

Isaiah 55:8-9 "For my thoughts are not your thoughts, neither are your ways my ways, saith the LORD. For as the heavens are higher than the earth, so are my ways higher than your ways, and my thoughts than your thoughts."

God loves us.  In the Old Testament, he made the nation of Israel to be his people.  But obedience was how they showed their love toward him.  It was because he loved them.  So many times, God forgave them and brought them back because he loved them.  We saw this begin with Adam and Eve.  It continued throughout history.

In the New Testament, we see the admonition to show our love by obeying.  In John 14:15, Jesus said, "If ye love me, keep my commandments."  Again, in John 14:23, "Jesus answered and said unto him, If a man love me, he will keep my words:"

Some people do not need boundaries with food; this is not their problem area.  For others of us, this is one of the ways God shows his love to us. He gives us guidelines for our food.   Because we know His ways are above our ways, we will obey.  If we trust God, we will do as he tells us.   Your mind will have to re-adjust, to think His thoughts, and not your own.

To be able to think God's thoughts, we need to know what his word says.  Choose a verse to use for meditation. It helps me to begin to memorize a scripture.  When I first started this, I would copy the verse into a reminder app on my phone and read it three times every time it came up on my phone.  I would have it come up seven times in a day.  Some of you may not need this much.  There are many ways to do this.  This suggestion is just something to get you started.

For right now, choose a scripture to memorize and meditate on it.  In a later chapter, we will cover other ways you can use the scriptures to change your thinking. This tool is often called the "renewing of the mind."

Here are a few scriptures to get you started. Looking at the ones in this chapter, Jeremiah 31:3 will remind you of God's great love for you.  Isaiah 55: 8 or 9, or both will tell you of how much greater God's wisdom is above yours.

Journaling questions:

1. What is your understanding of God's love for you? Write Jeremiah 31:3 in your journal.
2. Which verse are you going to begin memorizing?
3. What method will you use to help you with this? Do it.

# CHAPTER 3 - BOUNDARIES IN OUR LIVES

Imagine a cow in a field sticking her head through a barb wire fence to eat the grass on the other side of the fence. She is bleeding from the scratches on her neck from the barbed wire, and she doesn't care. She thinks the grass on the other side is greener and must be better. She doesn't understand why the farmer has put up a fence. She sees no danger in the trucks on the road just beyond the strip of grass she is trying to eat.

I first learned about boundaries when I was a little child. We lived in a house where the backyard went back to a river. It was near the mouth of the river that flowed into the Pacific Ocean. The river at that point was both deep and swift. There was a "sea wall" at the back of the property. This wall was a secure fence of logs, made much like a log house, only with the timbers in an upright position. It was to protect the land at the times the river got deep and overflowed the banks.

There were gates built into the sea wall in various places that could open up to get to the river edge. One of these gates was behind our house. I had strict instructions from my parents to never open or go through that gate. I was four years old and understood what those instructions meant. I also knew why it was dangerous.

One day the two neighbor kids, who were near my age, said, "Let's go through your gate and look at the river."

I said, "I'm not allowed to open the gate or go through it."

They said, "It's okay, the river is not up to the sea wall, it will be okay. We can just go through and see it and come back. Your Mom and Dad will not know."

I was a logical child; what they said sounded reasonable to me. I knew I was not to disobey my parents, but I also had a typical child's curiosity and wanted to go along with the other kids and have them like me. I agreed. Off the three of us went. We were not through the gate for more than a minute when I heard my father calling. "Judy, Judy, where are you?"

I knew I was caught. I had to go back. We all went back. My father knew I had disobeyed him. My father was so scared. He knew how easy it was for a little child of four to drown in that river. I knew I had disobeyed, and now I would be punished. I was. It was the worse spanking of my life, and I never forgot it.

No excuse I gave made any difference. "The neighbor kids wanted to go." "We were just looking." "The river wasn't high today." The boundary had been crossed, and I was to be punished.

I learned about boundaries in this true story.  I knew my father loved me.  I learned there were good reasons he gave me boundaries.

God is my heavenly father, and he cares about me.  There are good reasons God gives me boundaries.  Boundaries from God are for my good.

God gives boundaries in many areas of our lives.  When he gave the children of Israel the Ten Commandments, he added a lot of new limitations.  These had not only to do with their relationship with God, but with their relationship with other people.  Don't steal, don't commit adultery, don't kill, and many more.  We have no problem with these boundaries.  We understand the seriousness of the consequences.

One of the Ten Commandments has to do with having no other gods before the one true God.  In other teachings, we learn there is only one God.  In the world the Israelites lived in, many people worshipped other "things" and called them their gods.

Journal Questions:

1.      What are your thoughts on God giving you boundaries that have to do with your relationship with food?

2.      Was there a time when you let your love of food fill in for the love you should be giving to God?  Write about it.

3.	Write about a time when you let your love of food lead you to eat when you knew it was not right for you.

# CHAPTER 4 - IS FOOD A GOD FOR MY EMOTIONS?

Sometimes people go to food for comfort in stressful situations. I have done this.

When I was going to nursing school, it was stressful. I gained more than "the freshman five." I put on about 20 pounds over three years. Every time there was an exam coming, I would eat candy to get me through the studying. This situation was not the first time I had used food to calm my nerves or help get me through a tedious job.

Many years before I had learned that some foods gave a temporary feeling of comfort. I even introduced this to my husband, a person who had never overeaten.

We were going through a time when there were more bills than there was money to meet the need. Don was working a full-time job and two part-time jobs. I was home caring for our two children, but also doing occasional odd jobs and babysitting neighbor kids to try to get extra money. One night I could tell he was stressed. I told him, "Have some chocolate ice cream, it will make you feel better." So, he did, and it helped. Temporarily. False gods like food will only work temporarily. If we continue to misuse them, we reap the consequences of either extra weight, poor health, or both.

Some people go to other substances in their times of stress. Unfortunately, these other substances are usually addictive. It doesn't make food okay, just because it is not addictive. God did not make it to relieve stress. He made food for nourishment. Our creator made food to help our bodies grow and heal and repair themselves. He is a good God. He wanted us to enjoy food while we were doing our bodies' benefit; therefore, he made it taste good.

God wants to meet all our needs. Our God is a jealous god. Exodus 34:14 "For thou shalt worship no other god: for the LORD, whose name is Jealous, is a jealous God:" He does not want us going to things instead of going to Him.

What about the consequences of breaking the boundaries he has given us for our eating? It is well known that people who are overweight are at a much higher risk of health problems, especially if the person is inactive. I believe there is also a need God gives us for activity.

Many of you may doubt this right now. I used to be there too. Did God care about what I ate? Why would he care how much and whether I was overweight and in poor health? I was the one who put the food in my mouth. It was my elbow that bent my arm so I could get the fork to my mouth.  I took full responsibility for my actions and thought the remedy should also be my responsibility.  In a later chapter, I will discuss what changed my mind.

I also understand God no longer has specific boundaries regarding food for us.  He said he has made all foods clean and we may eat freely.   I also know many people maintain good health without ever having to pay attention to what or how much they eat.  For me, and possibly for you, it is not that way.  Some of us seem to use food for more than the nourishment our body needs to stay healthy.  For us, we need help.  We need guidelines.  In the next chapter, I will discuss the possible guidelines God may have for you individually.  For now, the purpose is to have you think about the possibility that God may have boundaries for you regarding food.

Journal questions:

1. Write about a time when you used food to relieve yourself from dealing with unwanted emotions?
2. What are some boundaries you have in your life in other areas?   Possible examples are these: Behavior with members of the opposite sex, in what clothing you wear, or in regards to another person's property.
3. Write about a time you let food occupy a position in your life that belonged to God.
4. Write about the possibility of having boundaries with food.

# CHAPTER 5 - MY INTRODUCTION TO FOOD BOUNDARIES

I began an explanation for food boundaries in Chapter One. This concept is fundamental, and I will use this chapter to do a more thorough explanation.

I was first introduced to food boundaries when I was very desperate to lose weight. I had just gone through an emotional roller coaster year. It is not that an emotional roller coaster is an excuse to overeat. It is to tell you about my story. Some people may relate.

In that year, I think I gained at least twenty more pounds. This poundage is above the twenty I had gained during nursing school.

Briefly, June - I was finishing nursing school and studying for the exam to get licensed as a registered nurse. I took the exam and passed it. In July, I began a new job. I loved my work as a registered nurse. A few weeks later, our middle son drowned. To deal with this deep grief, I ate to relieve the pain and gained ten pounds, or more, in a month. In December, my mother was diagnosed with a brain tumor and died three months later. January found me driving eight hours up to visit her every week. It was a lot of driving, and I used a lot of sweetened creamy coffee to stay awake. I had never had so many highs and so many lows, lower than low I had ever experienced, in less than twelve months. This tale is only part of the story of all that happened during those ten months. I was also twenty pounds heavier, added on to the twenty pounds I had gained in nursing school. Physically, I was miserable. I was at least forty pounds above any "normal" weight I had ever been. I turned to God for help.

I know God was there all the time. In all of the pressure and stress, I could barely pray. Others prayed for me. So many people prayed for me. I appreciated every prayer. I did not care what religion they came from; I welcomed all prayers. It was all I had. My prayers were full of fear and feelings of hopelessness.

My prayers were mostly just, "Help me, God." I knew he could use other's prayers to get me through this most difficult time. I never felt like he didn't care. I just didn't understand. I quoted from Job 1:21b, "the LORD gave, and the LORD hath taken away; blessed be the name of the LORD." I had a steady trust that He was there and would somehow make it work to my good. Romans 8:28 "And we know that all things work together for good to them that love God, to them who are the called according to his purpose." I appreciated this scripture but was so tired of hearing it when I could see nothing good possibly resulting. I was floundering in all these emotions. I felt so lost and desperate.

By the end of March, I was tired of the emotional roller coaster. I was ready to be done grieving.  I remembered when King David had quit grieving after his son died.  You can read the full story in Second Samuel chapter twelve, but what came to my memory was this part of verse 23 "can I bring him back again? I shall go to him, but he shall not return to me."

I laid aside the grief and began to seek God for an answer to the excess weight and the health problems it was causing.  My joints were aching; I woke up hurting; I knew I was snoring.  I was miserable.  None of the nursing uniforms I wore in nursing school fit, and I had to get new ones.  None of my regular clothes fit either.  I had a paycheck and had to spend it on getting new clothes. I had hoped to be able to pay off bills.

In my desperation, I continued to pray.  It seemed God comforted me and told me he would lead me to help.  I had gained and lost weight before by my own efforts.  I knew I could do it, but none of my usual diets were working.  I couldn't get myself to stick with anything. Everything I tried seemed to be another stressor.

God, ever a loving guide for me, led me to look for a scripturally based weight loss group.  I found a meeting advertised in the newspaper, and it fit in my schedule.  In relief, I went.  It promised so much hope I cried through most of the video introduction.  It was a program that used the boundaries of hunger and fullness.  It was a straightforward approach to weight loss using our natural hunger signals.  It also gave guidelines for those who had trouble discerning these signals.  It was simple enough I felt I could do it.  No measuring, no weighing foods, no trying to figure out what to eat, just eat what was there or what I wanted.  For me, it was what I needed.

I lost weight slowly and steadily at about one pound per week.  I was very encouraged.

It was in the mid-nineties, and God used it to begin my journey to freedom from the appetite for excess food.

There is one more Scripture passage I want to give before discussing food boundaries.

Psalm 16:5, "The LORD is the portion of mine inheritance and of my cup: thou maintainest my lot." Verse 6 "The lines are fallen unto me in pleasant places; yea, I have a goodly heritage."

In verse five, we see how the Lord is our inheritance, and in verse six, the lines have fallen in pleasant places.  I believe this means God is a generous God.  He has a good heritage for us.  He will not ask us to have boundaries for us that are going to make us miserable.  Not that our limits will please our fleshly desires, but they will be good for our bodies.  We will not be physically pained with God's boundaries.

Also, when God tells us his yoke is easy, and his burden is light, Matthew 11:30, this is not limited to how we feel when we first get salvation from sin.  I believe he would not have made us with a burden to bear that would be worse than what disobedience would be.

Our bodies are all different and react to foods differently. It is why I believe each of us needs to pray about what God wants us to use for food boundaries.

Journal time:

1. What food boundaries do you feel God leading you to use?
2. What, in your life, will make, or has made, you desperate enough to get away from the continual bondage to excess appetite?
3. Explain why you are desperate enough to make these into permanent changes.
4. If you still don't know what boundaries God is leading you to, spend time in earnest conversation with God about it today.

# CHAPTER 6 - POSSIBLE FOOD BOUNDARIES

God will help you find what works best for your body. He is our creator. Your creator knows your personality and your body. He knows what your weaknesses are and what your strengths are.

The teaching I first received that worked so well for me was to listen to my body as God had made it to lead me. Summarizing, these teachings are that God has given us a built-in way to know when to eat and when not to eat. They also taught us that this included our body, knowing what to eat and how much. For emotional and spiritual needs, we were to turn to God. Spiritual and emotional hunger is real, but it is not satisfied with food.

If a person paid close attention to their body, they would know when, what, and how much to eat. We feel physical hunger in our stomach. Emotional hunger will be in our minds, but not be giving a signal to our stomach. If we are just a person who likes a "sensation," and I have certainly experienced this, the desire for the sensation is often in our mind and maybe even in our mouth. I can "almost taste" whatever it is I think I am hungry for. Desiring a particular taste is not a bodily need.  This sensation is often more related to a feeling of anxiety.

The feeling in your stomach that indicates real physical hunger is sometimes an ache and sometimes a hollow feeling.  Some have an actual growl in their stomach, but not all.  To learn to feel a level of satisfaction is often more difficult.  From my experience, I cannot tell when I feel true satisfaction unless I have started at real physical hunger.

Listening to your body does work for many people.  It does not work for all people.  Some can never get it figured out for their body.  Some people need to have more structure because of their family obligations or other restrictions that make it not work. Other people may discover there are some foods their body is sensitive to and need to leave these foods out of their diets.

What is the alternative?

In the case of food sensitivities or allergies, they simply leave out the foods they are sensitive to and eat what they can enjoy when hungry.

For some, certain foods throw off their ability to know when they are no longer hungry.  These foods make it more difficult to sense when they have eaten enough once they begin.  One example of this is sugar.  Some people find they will crave more and more sugar if they have even a small amount.  For other people, it may be a high sodium starchy food.  You have to pay attention to your body and see how you react to these things. Everyone is different. I cannot tell you precisely what is going to work for you without asking a lot of questions.

Some people's lives require it to be more straightforward. For them to make a basic plan like "three meals a day and no seconds" is what works. For others, this would not work because they would pile their plates so high the first time their weight would go up steadily. Others have used it with great success.

Some people use a type of "Exchange Diet" because it works for them and their lifestyle. One example of this is Weight Watchers. Another example is the DASH Diet for lowering blood pressure.

One of the latest weight loss approaches is "intermittent fasting." Again, this is something many are find helpful, but some are not able to use it because they eat so much in the hours they are allowed to eat.

For you, it may not be any of these. Be sure it is something you seriously feel God leads you to.

One thing I know for sure is that if you are serious, God will hear a desperate heart and answer your prayer. He will lead you and guide you and give you boundaries that are workable for your life. He does care, and he will guide you. It will not be anything that includes using drugs or special supplements. It may be that your body will need some nutrients supplemented just because of an inability to absorb sufficient from natural foods. I also do not think it requires extra or expensive foods.  Your eating plan should be something very workable for your life.

One more thing.  We are going to ask God to lead us and guide us to boundaries with food that are going to be for the rest of our life.  The guidelines will not change when we get down to a healthy size.  It does not mean that you will never change your boundaries.  It means you are willing to have the boundaries you feel guided to, as a lifelong guideline.  In the beginning, you may not get a clear indication of what you should do.  In this case, choose one and continue to pray.  For some of us, our bodies change as we age, and our boundaries change as a result.

Journal time:

1. Have you prayed about the boundaries God would want you to use for the rest of your life?  If not, you must do this now.
2. Here are suggestions of things to think and journal about if you don't seem to get any direction.
   a. Do you get stressed if you have to keep track of how much you are eating?
   b. Does your family have regular mealtimes?
   c. Do you have food allergies?
   d. Do you know if foods that are highly sweet or very salty cause you to eat more than you need?
   e. Is there a "diet" that you had done before that was easy and simple for you to use?

3.  Looking at your answers to the above questions, what are the possible boundaries God is leading you to use?

# CHAPTER 7 - DOES GOD CARE ABOUT MY HEALTH?

Rom 12:1 "I beseech you therefore, brethren, by the mercies of God, that ye present your bodies a living sacrifice, holy, acceptable unto God, which is your reasonable service."

Rom 12:2 "And be not conformed to this world: but be ye transformed by the renewing of your mind, that ye may prove what is that good, and acceptable, and perfect, will of God."

Psalm 139:14 "I will praise thee; for I am fearfully and wonderfully made: marvellous are thy works; and that my soul knoweth right well."

God has made our bodies.  He made our bodies to heal themselves or protect themselves from diseases most of the time.  I believe God cares if we take care of what he has given us.  I have to appreciate the body given to me. My body is his gift to me.

I also believe there is something I can do to take care of myself.  I realize my food and my weight affect my health. Diseases linked to overeating and conditions related to inactivity are atherosclerosis, heart disease, hypertension, cancer, strokes, Type II diabetes, fatty liver disease, and heart attacks.  These may not be diseases you have ever seen in your families.  For me, it is scary; almost all of them are in my family.  If there is anything I can do to avoid them, I feel it is my responsibility to do so.

As Christians, what is our goal in life?  I want to reach people with the gospel.  I want to teach people about the Bible.  I want to share with others the changes Jesus can make in our lives.  I want to live awhile longer and continue doing what God wants me to do.

God gives us a desire to live.  The longer we are alive, the longer we can work for him.

Journal Time:

1.  What are your goals for your health?
2.  Why do you think God cares about our health?
3.  Do you think to present our bodies to him to use, as it states in Romans 12:1, has to do with the physical body or just the spiritual part of you?
4.  What do you think is meant by this scripture? Psalm 139:14 "I will praise thee; for I am fearfully and wonderfully made: marvellous are thy works; and that my soul knoweth right well."

# CHAPTER 8 - WHO CARES HOW HEALTHY I AM?

The nurse went out of the room to let the doctor know I was ready for my annual exam.  I saw she had left my patient chart sitting on the table next to the exam table.  I reached over and picked it up.  I began to read, "This obese woman…"  I don't remember what it said after that; just that shocked me.  It brought to my attention that I was not 'just a little overweight.'  My blood pressure was high, and my cholesterol was high.  It was not to be ignored; I needed to do something about it.

Most of us know at least some of the health effects of being overweight.  When you have a friend or relative who has died from the results of obesity, it can hit you hard.

Young people often ignore the risks in their health habits.  They believe the end of life is so far away.  A young person may feel there is a lot of time to change their practices. When you reach middle age, or even in the mid-thirties, it begins to get your attention.

One of the problems with health information is that it changes. It is twofold. There are discoveries made yearly in healthcare and science. The other half of it is false information. "News" without any research behind it, or "news" based on only one study.

Because of this, I have referred to the Centers for Disease Control for information. I do not want to be a purveyor of false information. There are already enough of those. I do not need to make things up to tell you that obesity is harmful to your health. Here is where you can look for information that is the current news.

The CDC website: https://www.cdc.gov/healthyweight/effects/index.html

It is possible to be very healthy and still be overweight. This possibility doesn't change the need to take care of our bodies and prevent problems. It also doesn't mean you will need to lose a lot of weight to be healthy.

When I was a young adult, I began to read a lot of books on proper nutrition. When I started to have children, it stirred a renewed interest in nutritious food. I wanted to do the best I could for them. Unfortunately, my human love for all things yummy, this lust of the flesh for foods that delighted my taste buds, often interfered with me eating only foods that were good for me. It also interfered with feeding my family only the foods that were good for them. Although if you ask my children, all they will recall is the year we all went off of sugar, and they felt like the most deprived children in the USA.

As the years went by, I realized that the "food rules" and the nutrition guidelines recommended switched about as often as the president of the USA and the surgeon general changed.  I had also lived in Canada and saw their eating guidelines change, as well.  Then there were all the books put out by the health food fanatics.  Most had admirable goals of helping mothers raise healthy children.  But from them, I could see the advice swing from "eat more protein" to "too much protein is hard on the kidneys."  Then "eat more whole grains" to "gluten from grains causes health problems."  Another went from "eat only healthy oils" to "eat all the fat you want."  What was a mother to think?

Not only that, but I was a daughter of a mother who didn't know very much about nutrition other than "make sure there is at least one fruit and one vegetable in your diet every day."  My father believed every new health fad that came by.  And we tried out everything he was thinking was the answer to a long life—everything from eating fresh yogurt to drinking goat's milk.  I am sure there were more that are not coming to mind, but if someone convinced him, we tried it.  He added, but never subtracted any of the things he ate that were not good for him.

As an adult, I worried about my parent's health.  I could see how overweight and inactive they seemed to be.  I was sure they were going to kill themselves with their bad habits.  I worried about things that made no difference, like how much coffee they drank.  Their coffee was so weak it was like weak tea. In the 1970s, caffeine was considered harmful. No one knew what else could be in the coffee bean. Recent research has shown there are antioxidants in coffee, and what they were drinking was insignificant. I also worried about the amount of animal fat they were eating. Then there was their bologna and wieners, the processed meats—so many concerns. I would try to educate them, but it made little difference. They were the parents and felt they knew more than I did.

My children loved it when my parents visited because my father always had candy in the car when he drove. He would eat it while he drove to keep himself alert. The kids knew where to find the sugar.

Now, as adults, my children worry about the health of their father and me. They do care that we stay healthy. They saw me lose my parents when they were comparatively young. Losing your parents when they are young is hard. It is especially hard when you think they could have lived longer if they had taken care of themselves.


Journal questions:

1. To what degree do you care if the people in your life are healthy or not?
2. How much concern do you, or did you, want your parents to be healthy?

3. What have your children ever said to you about wanting you to stay healthy?
4. Do you have a family history of any of the diseases that can be made worse by obesity?  If so, how concerned are you about getting these?
5. What other health concerns do you have because of your weight?

# CHAPTER 9 - WE KNOW BETTER; WHY DON'T WE DO BETTER?

The majority of women in First World countries have been on a "diet" at some time in their life.  You have probably been one of them.  You have been able to lose weight.  Many of us have lost the same 10, 20, 30, or 40 pounds over and over again.  I have.  There are multiple numbers of ways to lose weight.  Keeping it off is the problem.

Knowing how to lose weight is not the main problem. Knowing how to eat according to a reasonable eating plan is not the problem.  Consistency is the problem.  The thing is, we can be consistent with so many things.  There are so many things that don't even tempt us.

For myself, I could attend church, school, work, anything I was committed to, without ever missing a day.  I had read my Bible for years on end without missing a day, and prayer time was a regular habit for years.  We brush our teeth and take a shower every day.  You probably have these and many other practices that are very consistent for you.  Knowing how to be consistent is not the problem.  It was knowing how to be consistent with eating the way God had directed me.  There was my problem, my hang-up.  There were many "tricks" I used to help myself stay consistent when I went "on a diet."  They were of little long-term value.

Journal questions:

1. Write about other times when you had success with weight loss.
2. In what other areas of your life have you been able to be consistent?
3. What circumstances came up that kept you from being consistent with your eating plan?
4. If you want to lose weight, what is your biggest reason?  It is beneficial to know WHY you are making changes.

# CHAPTER 10 - DO YOU NEED HELP?

I have kept my weight in about a 10-pound range and my health stable for a few years now. You can do the same. Others have helped me. I heard someone recently say that God made people to "live in community." I hadn't thought about that before, but I realized I do believe that. He gave us a desire to work together with others. It begins when we are born into a family. That is our first community. When we become Christians, we become a part of the family of God. The church is a community. Life goes better when we have help. We will enjoy life more if we help others.

Let us look at some scriptures.

Hebrews 10:24-25 "And let us consider one another to provoke unto love and to good works: Not forsaking the assembling of ourselves together, as the manner of some is; but exhorting one another: and so much the more, as ye see the day approaching."

1Peter 5:5 "Likewise, ye younger, submit yourselves unto the elder. Yea, all of you be subject one to another, and be clothed with humility: for God resisteth the proud, and giveth grace to the humble."

1Corinthians 12:28 "And God hath set some in the church, first apostles, secondarily prophets, thirdly teachers, after that miracles, then gifts of healings, helps, governments, diversities of tongues."

If we are trying to do something on our own and failing, consider whether you need another to "provoke you to good works:" or perhaps you need to submit to another who knows more about what you are needing.  We can all be "subject one to another."  It all requires humility.  I am thankful God promises grace to the humble.  I am not perfect and rely so much on the grace and mercy of God. Without being a part of the larger body of Christ, the church, we would not have all of the ministries available to us.

For myself, I would do well when I had a group leader, or a personal accountability partner to help me.  When I did not have one of these, I would flounder.  I could do good for a while if I were doing an online lesson.  When the class was over, I would be off track again.  It didn't matter how strong my reasons for wanting to be in good health were.  The flesh was weak, and I needed God and human support to keep going consistently for a long time.

When I finally found an online (Facebook) group that was available every day, all year, it was a lifesaver.  Sometimes I did not do the class they were doing, sometimes I did another study or even just read through a book on my own, but I would make myself accountable to them every day.  I was also assigned a couple of ladies to be accountability partners with; we all needed help one as much as another.  I needed someone who was always there to encourage me and give me the support I needed.

Eventually, I was able to be a leader.  Now I can be a person giving others the support they need.  God led me slowly by slowly, step by step. As long as I stayed committed, he was faithful to keep leading me on with the help of good people he put into my life.

Journal questions:

1. When you tried losing weight independently with no support, how successful were you?  Are you still using the same method and staying consistent?
2. Have you been part of a weight loss group?  How successful were you when you had support?
3. Have you been able to be a support to another?

# CHAPTER 11 - YOUR BODY, GOD'S TEMPLE

Do you believe your body is the temple of God?  If you have the Holy Spirit, you know the Bible says in I Corinthians 3:16, "Know ye not that ye are the temple of God, and that the Spirit of God dwelleth in you?"  Verse 17 says, "If any man defile the temple of God, him shall God destroy; for the temple of God is holy, which temple ye are."  And verse 18, "Let no man deceive himself."

And then in I Corinthians 6:19 "What? know ye not that your body is the temple of the Holy Ghost which is in you, which ye have of God, and ye are not your own?" verse 20 "For ye are bought with a price: therefore glorify God in your body, and in your spirit, which are God's."  This application is controversial to some people.  They say it is referring only to the sin of fornication, which it mentions in the verse before it.  Perhaps, if it is a sin that can affect your body and spirit, then it is applicable.  The principle applies.  I have no doubt overeating affects the body.  I also know that being overweight can cause some negative emotions, which no doubt affects the spirit of a person.

These verses are convicting to me if I am doing something that is not taking care of God's temple.  I want to be a good steward of what God has given me.  He has put my body in my care.  He has made it and entrusted it to me. How should I treat God's dwelling place?  Of course, I should not allow it to sin.  I want to take decent care of it. I want to be kind to it.  I want to move it enough to keep it healthy.  I want to feed it enough to keep it nourished.  I want to keep it looking holy.  We serve a holy God.  I must keep my mind and soul pure.

It is interesting to me to note that all of these scriptures are in I and II Corinthians.  These are letters Paul found necessary to write to a church he loved.  But he had to address its carnality.  When I am overeating, I am getting carnal.  I am feeding the lusts of the flesh.  That is all there is to it.

Another scripture I want to look at in I Corinthians is in chapter 10, verse 31 "Whether therefore ye eat, or drink, or whatsoever ye do, do all to the glory of God."  I realize he had been addressing eating things served to idols and whether they should partake of them or not. But since it says "whatsoever ye do," including eating or drinking, think of this, is your eating and drinking to the glory of God?

On the same line of thought, look at Colossians 3:17 "And whatsoever ye do in word or deed, do all in the name of the Lord Jesus, giving thanks to God and the Father by him." Again, we see this word, *whatsoever* we do in word or deed.  A lot of people made light of the WWJD movement a few years back.  But what about the verse that says, "Do all in the name of the Lord Jesus?"   "All" is pretty broad.  If applied to all we do, it covers all we do, including our food consumption.

He will not leave me nor forsake me.  He will be there to help me in what I do and how I care for it.  In Hebrews 13:5 we are told, "Let your conversation be without covetousness; and be content with such things as ye have: for he hath said, I will never leave thee, nor forsake thee." I know that if I am willing to be content with what God gives me, he will give me what I need.

Jesus taught in his parables that God expects us to be good stewards of the gifts he gives us.  My body, even as it ages, and with its deficits, is a gift from God.

Journal Questions:

1. Why do you think God cares about how you care for your body?
2. Journal about the responsibility you feel to care for your body now, after reading the above scriptures.
3. Can you find other scripture that shows how God cares and wants to help you take care of your body?

# CHAPTER 12 - WHAT THE BIBLE SAYS

Does the Bible have anything to say about our food or our eating?  At one time, I did not think it did.  I had attended church from the Sunday after my mother brought me home from the hospital, and I did not recall hearing any teaching or preaching on eating.  I thought everything addressed in the Bible had been taught in our church. From somewhere I had heard that gluttony was a sin, but believed the definition someone told me.  I had heard the meaning of gluttony was when the person ate so much, they threw up and then went back to eat some more.  Of course, that is the definition of gorge and purge or bulimia. I also heard some more formal churches taught it was one of the seven deadly sins.  I knew I did not throw up after eating.  But my conscience reminded me, "after a Thanksgiving meal or other large celebratory meal, you are so stuffed you burp some up." I would reason within myself, "Surely, that isn't the same."

One day I looked for the word gluttony in a comprehensive Bible concordance. Obviously, I was a little concerned about it since I was looking it up.  I couldn't find the word "gluttony" in the concordance.  In relief, I decided the Bible didn't address it. "It must be one of those sins they made up," I thought.  I didn't look any further at that time.

 In the late 1980s and early 1990s, when Christian writers began to address the issue of overeating, I cautiously looked into the scriptures they were using.  Then I began to pay closer attention.  When my weight ballooned up, I got more serious about looking for it, but could never maintain the conviction that overeating was a sin.  I saw some very spiritual people who were extremely overweight.  I saw leaders in our church who were overweight, some by a little, and some by much more.  I could not figure it out.

I knew people who had received the victory over alcoholism, drug abuse, and all kinds of deadly sins when they got saved.  No one ever gave a testimony of being free from wanting to overeat.  Sometimes these people's weight went up as they ate more and more after quitting alcohol, drugs, or cigarettes.  The questions in my mind were more and more conflicted.

One thing these people who had overcome overeating had in common was their faith in the truth of the word of God.  Even if they didn't understand everything, they had a strong belief in the truth of what they understood. Was there something in the Bible I was missing?

Meanwhile, I read the testimonies of Christians who had overcome the desire to overeat with the use of Bible scriptures.  I felt defeated.  How could these people have that kind of victory when I did not?   They talked about how they spoke to God about their food issues, and he had answered them.  It was not something I had ever done.  I began to seek God and ask him to speak to me. The more I prayed about it and asked for his help, the more answers he gave me.  I learned that he spoke to me through his word most of the time.  Other times I would receive a gentle nudge in my spirit to think about something in a new way.  I realized that the better I got to know Jesus, the more I would hear from him.  The more I asked him to lead me and guide me, the more he answered.

I had long had a habit of reading through the Bible in a year.  This practice meant I read every day.  One year I decided I was going to try to write down some of the verses that applied to eating and food.  The first thing I noticed was that the first sin was someone eating something God said not to eat.  It wasn't someone using a drug or alcohol.  It was food!

I found several things in the Proverbs.   Often the overeating was linked with overuse of alcohol or drunkenness.  As if it fell in the same category.

Look at this from Proverbs 23 – verse 1 "When thou sittest to eat with a ruler, consider diligently what is before thee:" verse 2 "And put a knife to thy throat, if thou be a man given to appetite." Verse 3 "Be not desirous of his dainties: for they are deceitful meat."  I asked myself, "Am I a person 'given to appetite?'" Sometimes I have been.  I was mainly given to it when there were foods available that I didn't get often.  The "dainties" were not necessarily good for people's nutrition.  What if those dainties had been sweets and chocolate?  Oh, my, I would have been desiring them so much.  So much.  I could see how these verses applied to me and my eating habits.

Now here is another in Proverbs 23 that is about food. We see it linked with drunkenness. Verse 20 "Be not among winebibbers; among riotous eaters of flesh:" and verse 21 "For the drunkard and the glutton shall come to poverty: and drowsiness shall clothe a man with rags."  The drunkard and the glutton both have the same problem. Thinking about the phrase "riotous eaters of meat" brought to mind how happy or excited people had been when there was a potluck after church.  Guilt struck me. I was probably more excited about the deserts, and I sure wasn't going to be the last in line.

Looking into the New Testament, we see more.  I Peter 4:3 says, "For the time past of our life may suffice us to have wrought the will of the Gentiles, when we walked in lasciviousness, lusts, excess of wine, revellings, banquetings, and abominable idolatries:"  Verse 4, "Wherein they think it strange that ye run not with them to the same excess of riot, speaking evil of you:" Looking at the Strong's definition, most of those words speak of some form of wild partying.  Excesses and drunkenness.

Eating to excess is not listed among the works of the flesh in Paul's writing.  But when we look at the actions of the Spirit in Galatians chapter 5 verse 22, we see "But the fruit of the Spirit is love, joy, peace, longsuffering, gentleness, goodness, faith," verse 23 "Meekness, temperance: against such there is no law." Verse 24 "And they that are Christ's have crucified the flesh with the affections and lusts."  Verse 25 "If we live in the Spirit, let us also walk in the Spirit."  Temperance means moderation.  A standard definition in the 20th Century was that temperance meant no alcohol.  It doesn't mean temperance is limited to alcohol.

In Philippians, Paul says in chapter four, verse 5 – "Let your moderation be known unto all men."  Moderation means no excesses.  How would some of our fellowships change if we practiced restraint?  How many potlucks lead to excesses?  Many came to the potlucks at our church and ate in moderation.  It was easy to see those who had a problem with controlling the lust of their flesh for excess food.  I was among them.  My plate could hardly hold what I was getting.  I wanted to try everything.  It was a shame.

All "you can eat" buffets were another big problem. When I was breaking free of this bondage to the lusts of my appetite, I hated going to buffets.  I can't say I love them now, but at least I am not so afraid of going overboard out of my food boundaries.

One more scripture that stood out to me was this one in Philippians chapter three verse 18 "(For many walk, of whom I have told you often, and now tell you even weeping, that they are the enemies of the cross of Christ:" verse 19 "Whose end is destruction, whose God is their belly, and whose glory is in their shame, who mind earthly things.)"  I know this could mean not only the actual belly in a person but also simply their selfish, self-centered desires or their appetites in not only food.  It also convicts me to see that their glory was in their shame.  How many times had I joked about the "Christian sin" of eating?  Or joked, making light of the gorging done at a meal?  When someone stands up in one of our congregations and says something about "one thing we know how to do is eat;" I am ashamed.  It is glorying in our shame.

Multiple scriptures spoke to my heart since looking at this subject Biblically.  To me, the lusts and desires of the flesh can be associated with overeating.  Fornication, adultery, and drunkenness are all lusts repeated and well known by Bible-reading people. Appetite for excess food doesn't seem to be explicitly mentioned in the New Testament.  As a human, though, I know this lust.  It is a lust for more than I need—this lust for something God has so graciously supplied to meet our need for nourishment.

There is no limit from God on the 'what' of our food.  It is our heart and health that should guide us.  In I Corinthians six verse 12 it says, "All things are lawful unto me, but all things are not expedient: all things are lawful for me, but I will not be brought under the power of any."  Have you ever felt you were under the power of some food? Especially something that was not necessary for life, like sugar or candy or ice cream, or cake?  Or something salty like chips?  Often this will happen when you have seen them in a picture or smelled them.  Or perhaps, if you had a few earlier and your appetite keeps telling you how good it was, and you want more even though you know you don't need it and aren't hungry?  Or have you started eating something and can't get yourself to stop, although you know you have had more than you need?

Journaling Questions

1. When was the first time you felt convicted by scripture in regards to your eating?
2. What scriptures spoke to your heart?
3. Is it circumstances, a particular food, or both that gives you a hard time stopping when you know you are eating more than you know your body needs?
4. Journal about these situations and what it is that is causing the overeating.
5. Are you ready to set some boundaries for your eating?  Begin today, if you haven't already, to set some simple boundaries on your food consumption.  Examples are - to not eat until hungry and stop eating when no longer hungry, or to limit your eating to three meals a day, all when seated at the table.

# CHAPTER 13 - MIND RENEWAL TOOLS

As I was learning how to let go of this grip the lust for food had on my mind, I learned I needed a transformation in my thinking regarding food. The way I thought of food was so lustful. I would see it and lust for a taste because it looked like it would taste good. Maybe the sensation on my palate was what I lusted for. I would consider the cost, and I wasn't thinking about the damage to my body, only to my wallet. If I thought I could afford it, I bought it. It didn't matter if it was food with ingredients of no benefit to my body. I purchased the "sensation." Many times, I was disappointed. So disappointed. It was looking like one thing and tasting like another. That is how it goes with lusts. You think you are getting something so amazing, but if it is not in God's plan, it is so wrong.

I also had a problem with wanting to eat more than I needed. It continues to be a struggle from time to time. It is especially true when the food is "good for me." Nothing is "good for me" if my body doesn't need it. My mind will fool me temporarily into thinking that I shouldn't waste it because it is so full of nutrients.  This thinking is wrong.  If it is more than I need right now, I can save it.  The waste is to eat it now.

There are multiple ways of eating when and what we don't need.  I found I was not the only one who went through this.  Many, many people went through the very same temptations.  Fortunately, I began to learn ways to change my thinking to thinking more like Jesus would want me to think.

The Bible says in Romans 12:1 & 2 says, "I beseech you therefore, brethren, by the mercies of God, that ye present your bodies a living sacrifice, holy, acceptable unto God, which is your reasonable service. And be not conformed to this world: but be ye transformed by the renewing of your mind, that ye may prove what is that good, and acceptable, and perfect, will of God."

I will share the resources from which I learned.  They are far better at explaining the specifics than I am.   I recommend these.

The first resources I came across were by author Barb Ravelings.   She has a book on mind renewal, *"The Renewing of the Mind Project."*  This book was full of a lot of useful information and opened my mind to a way to change my thinking using God's word.  To deal directly with eating, though, is another resource I use.  It is her book or app called *"I Deserve A Donut."*  This little book has questions to use that bring your thinking in alignment with what is right for you.  It will also give you scriptures to go with almost every situation you come across in this ongoing temptation to overeat.

Another book that covers even more ways to renew your mind using scripture is a book by Sophia Tucker called *"Renewing of the Mind 101."* If you are not familiar with mind renewal techniques, this book gives you an excellent overall summary of many with easy "How To" directions in each section. I also learned some from reading Dr. Carolyn Leaf's works. Her books explain the science behind mind renewal.

I learned the scripture memorization techniques from international speaker, Melani Shock. She was teaching at a seminar I attended. The first verses I memorized were some she recommended. Joshua 1:8,9 – "This book of the law shall not depart out of thy mouth; but thou shalt meditate therein day and night, that thou mayest observe to do according to all that is written therein: for then thou shalt make thy way prosperous, and then thou shalt have good success. Have not I commanded thee? Be strong and of a good courage; be not afraid, neither be thou dismayed: for the LORD thy God is with thee whithersoever thou goest." We see here that the purpose of scripture is to meditate on it. Then we will have good success. That is what we all want.

Journaling questions:

1.    Which of these mind renewal tools have you used?

2.      Have you been using any of the memory or scripture meditation examples I have given?

3.      What have you found helpful?

4.      Which will you use today?

# CHAPTER 14 - RELEASED FROM BONDAGE

It is not unusual to feel that your thoughts are in bondage when it comes to an appetite for too much food.  Have you said or heard someone say, "I just crave it," "I can't help it," or "I couldn't resist it?"  They, or you, or I, feel in bondage.  We feel bound to do what we know is not beneficial for us.

In Romans, Paul said in chapter 7:14-25, "For we know that the law is spiritual: but I am carnal, sold under sin. For that which I do I allow not: for what I would, that do I not; but what I hate, that do I. If then I do that which I would not, I consent unto the law that it is good. Now then it is no more I that do it, but sin that dwelleth in me. For I know that in me (that is, in my flesh,) dwelleth no good thing: for to will is present with me; but how to perform that which is good I find not. For the good that I would I do not: but the evil which I would not, that I do. Now if I do that I would not, it is no more I that do it, but sin that dwelleth in me. I find then a law, that, when I would do good, evil is present with me. For I delight in the law of God after the inward man: But I see another law in my members, warring against the law of my mind, and bringing me into captivity to the law of sin which is in my members. O wretched man that I am! who shall deliver me from the body of this death? I thank God through Jesus Christ our Lord. So then with the mind I myself serve the law of God; but with the flesh the law of sin."

That is a lot of fighting between the desires of the flesh and the will of God.  For now, let us look at "that which I do I allow not: for what I would, that do I not; but what I hate, that do I."  then the phrase, "bringing me into captivity to the law of sin which is in my members." And then, "who shall deliver me."  When I was fighting the lusts of the flesh, and it seemed like I was in bondage to this craving for more food than I needed, God showed me an illustration of bondage in the Old Testament.

When Moses had reached the end of his ministry and brought the Israelites to the Jordan River, he gave them over to Joshua to lead into Canaan.  Canaan was a beautiful land, a land flowing with milk and honey, by their description.  God promised the land to them, and they were to go in and conquer it all.

In Deuteronomy, Moses told them all of the blessings they would receive if they obeyed and conquered all and did not serve the gods of the nations where they were going. Moses also told them all of the curses that would come about when they disobeyed.  God knew before they went in that they would sometimes disobey him.

Deuteronomy 31:16-18 "And the LORD said unto Moses, Behold, thou shalt sleep with thy fathers; and this people will rise up, and go a whoring after the gods of the strangers of the land, whither they go to be among them, and will forsake me, and break my covenant which I have made with them. Then my anger shall be kindled against them in that day, and I will forsake them, and I will hide my face from them, and they shall be devoured, and many evils and troubles shall befall them; so that they will say in that day, Are not these evils come upon us, because our God is not among us? And I will surely hide my face in that day for all the evils which they shall have wrought, in that they are turned unto other gods."

We see right soon that they made a covenant with another nation who fooled them into thinking that they were a nation from far away.  In Joshua chapter nine, we see where the Gibeonites fooled them into thinking they were from a long way off and agreed to be their servants if they would not go to war against them.  The Gibeonites were fearful of them, and rightly so because the Israelites had already conquered several kingdom/cities.

The Gibeonites were not the only ones who were not driven out or wholly destroyed.  By the time Joshua was coming to the end of his life, they had several cities not yet conquered.  They were satisfied to just live amongst them, and when they could, put them to tribute.

Joshua 17:12-13 "Yet the children of Manasseh could not drive out the inhabitants of those cities; but the

Canaanites would dwell in that land. Yet it came to pass, when the children of Israel were waxen strong, that they put the Canaanites to tribute; but did not utterly drive them out."

In Joshua 23, the Israelites receive instructions to go in and finish conquering.  God promises he will help them. The area is divided between the tribes.  Joshua tells them in verses 5-7, "And the LORD your God, he shall expel them from before you, and drive them from out of your sight; and ye shall possess their land, as the LORD your God hath promised unto you. Be ye therefore very courageous to keep and to do all that is written in the book of the law of Moses, that ye turn not aside therefrom to the right hand or to the left; That ye come not among these nations, these that remain among you; neither make mention of the name of their gods, nor cause to swear by them, neither serve them, nor bow yourselves unto them:"

They hear about the dangers.  They receive instructions on what to do and why.

Joshua 23:11-13 "Take good heed therefore unto yourselves, that ye love the LORD your God. Else if ye do in any wise go back, and cleave unto the remnant of these nations, even these that remain among you, and shall make marriages with them, and go in unto them, and they to you: Know for a certainty that the LORD your God will no more drive out any of these nations from before you; but they shall be snares and traps unto you, and scourges in your sides, and thorns in your eyes, until ye perish from off this good land which the LORD your God hath given you."

It is in this illustration I see a comparison to us when we come to God, and he asks us to give up everything and serve him.  We agree, we go to war with the enemy of our soul, and we repent of all our sins.  As it goes on, we are living victorious and feeling so good.  Then something comes along and makes a treaty with us.  "Let me just do this, and I won't bother you."  The flesh begins to bargain.  We may or may not even be aware of the bargain going on between our flesh and spirit.  It says, "I will give up the alcohol, I will give up the illegal drugs.  Those are not good for me anyway, and everyone knows it.  But this appetite for excess food, that's not so bad."  I have heard alcoholics make the excuse that they need the extra carbohydrates to keep from craving alcohol.  They have traded one high for another.  It is not quite as damaging, at least not in the short run.  Some have given up cigarettes and taken up compulsive eating of candy—same excuse.

What is God saying?  When we leave some of these things in our lives, there is a risk we will begin to serve them as a god.  Then we do not love God with all our soul, heart, and mind.  Instead of letting God conquer our excess appetite for food, also, we think we will "put it under tribute" or "make it a servant."  This commitment is hard to maintain.  If the appetites of the flesh are not conquered, they will arise again and take control of the body.

Journal Questions

1. From what forms of sinful bondage has God freed you?
2. How possible is it that God can do the same for you with food?
3. About what type of things have you ever made a bargain with God?  Did any have to do with what and how much food you will eat?
4. How have you justified your overeating?
5. What lies do you tell yourself about how you can keep it under control without following God's leading?

# CHAPTER 15 - "WHAT?  I'M NOT AN EMOTIONAL EATER."

"I could always tell when you were going through a difficult time, Mom; your weight was going up."

Daughters can be so honest.  They know you love them. Sometimes they notice things about you that you don't even see.  "Me, an emotional eater? I didn't think so."  I thought about it, but I said, "Really?  Oh, my! Wow!" "Maybe a little bit," I thought, but maybe it was more than just a little bit.  I recalled I had introduced my husband to the theory that you would feel better when worried if you ate a little (or a lot of) chocolate ice cream.

I began to observe myself.  The day was stressful at work; I knew who had dishes of chocolate candies on their desks.  I was happy to find an excuse.  "Chocolate is a mood booster.  It's good for you, plus it is supposed to be good for your heart."  Never mind the fact that the information was about very dark chocolate in small amounts.  It did not mean the available milk chocolate.

Another thing I did when my day had been stressful was bake.  Then I would eat.  Cookies were my favorite because it didn't take long to get them from raw ingredients to baked and ready to eat. Twenty minutes, ready, relax. A cake took too long. Although, if I made the frosting right away, I could have a spoon full of that while I waited for the cake to bake. Then I would eat more, and more and more. It never stopped with one or two cookies or one spoon of frosting.

Why did I turn to food to relieve anxiety, feeling sorry for myself, frustration, anger, sorrow? Yes, I was an emotional eater. I had forgotten about all those things. When I grieved, I ate so much I gained at least 10 pounds the first month and ten more in the following four months. Yes, I remembered that. When I had a high pressure, busy work schedule, I gained weight. I don't know how much. A lot. At least an additional 20 pounds. When I had an unexpected pregnancy, I added at least 20 pounds more than I needed. With all of my planned babies, I only gained what I needed. Afterward, I was fairly quickly back to a healthy weight. With that fourth, though, it was ridiculous. I used the excuse that the midwife thought I was having twins. Maybe the midwife thought I was having twins because I was gaining so much weight. Now there is circular thinking for you. I only had one baby. After that experience, all of her clients suspected of having twins had to get an ultrasound.

My daughter's observations were correct. I was an emotional eater. When I ate because of the emotions I was having, it lessened the strength of the feeling. For a few minutes, maybe a few hours, I would be relieved of the feelings I didn't want to have.  I wondered what it would be like if I let myself feel the emotion.  I was determined to change, so I again observed myself.  When I felt worried about driving in heavy traffic or having to drive a long way, I would have a bag of candies in the car to "Keep me awake."  That was a good excuse, but it also relieved the boredom.  I hated feeling bored.  I still hate that feeling.  Eating, tasting, getting an oral sensation, is more fun.

I had to learn there were other things I could do to stay alert while driving.  Eating is not the only thing I can do when I drive.

When I was frustrated or anxious about a situation, or worried about something at work, I began to let myself feel the feeling.  Number one, I didn't die from feeling the emotion.  Number two, I learned to see what the Bible had to say about that emotion and how to deal with it.  I prayed a lot more.

My old way was to tell God whatever it was that was troubling me, but then put the burden right back onto myself.  The turmoil was still in my soul.  I had to learn to go to God with it right away.  And do it again if necessary, over and over again.

Some of the things I learned in this were how I could learn to think God's thoughts on these matters.  Refer back to chapter 13 for the mind renewal tools.  I have found using the "Think on Model" from Sophia Tuckers book *Mind*

*Renewal 101*, and Barb Ravelings *I Deserve A Donut*, in the section dealing with emotions to be most helpful.

Ephesians 4:22-23, "And be renewed in the spirit of your mind; And that ye put on the new man, which after God is created in righteousness and true holiness."

Questions for journaling:

1. How effective has emotional eating been for you?
2. What emotions do you find most challenging for you?
3. What is the worst thing that will happen if you allow yourself to feel the emotions instead of covering them with eating?
4. What is your experience with giving God your emotions?
5. Some stressors cannot be removed and must be accepted.  It does not mean we have to eat to deal with them.  What happens when you accept the emotion and don't eat or do anything to cover it?
6. Which of the mind renewal tools will you use today when you have to deal with your emotions?

# CHAPTER 16 – DISCERNMENT: WHAT AM I HUNGRY FOR?

I needed to learn to discern between hunger from the body and hunger from the soul. When I was dealing with emotions that made me want to eat, I could often convince myself that I was hungry.

There is a difference between the two. The problem is learning to discern between the two hungers. First, I will cover how to tell when you are physically hungry. Body hunger is felt in the stomach. The physical stomach starts right below your sternum, and it curves around and beneath the ribs. It is covered a little by the ribs on both sides, but it mostly is to your right. When you feel a feeling of hunger, it is in this area. It may be a pain. It may be an empty hollow feeling, or it may be a crampy feeling.

Sometimes it is a feeling of weakness or a sudden drop in energy. Some people think their blood sugar is falling when they are suddenly weak. It is probably not the case. Blood sugar may drop a little and contribute to the feeling, but it is rare for it to fall to a dangerous level.

When it is hunger, it is not dangerous if you have to wait to eat.

The highest risk when you get over hungry is to overeat then.  The solution to this is to be aware and be careful.  Slow down and eat slowly.  It will be fine.  Very few people have a diagnosis of "low blood sugar," which is a medical condition.  These people need to follow the doctor's instructions.  For the remainder of us, we need to use the self-control we get from God as part of the fruit of the Spirit.  The more you nourish the fruit of the Spirit, the stronger and healthier it will be.

When you have "emotional hunger," it will be different. You will feel such an urgency to eat.  It comes on suddenly, and you may feel it in any part of the body.  If it is a "hunger" perceived in the mouth, drooling, or a craving for a favorite food, it is not physical hunger. Thoughts of food often trigger this sensation.  These can come from looking at the actual food or even photos of food.  It is vital for me to not stare at pictures of food.  I had to throw out and discontinue subscriptions to food magazines.  The photos were dangerous to my mind.  I also stopped subscription to many of my "food" authors from whom I received emails.  I also quit reading cookbooks.  I still use cookbooks, but only as needed.  I still have a few email subscriptions, but these are very limited.  If I find they are tripping me up, I know I can also discontinue these.

Another thing I did was start scrolling right past pictures of plates on Facebook or Instagram.  I will rarely post a photo like that.  I may post a photo of a great meal that is culturally interesting.  I don't want to trip others up.

This hunger of the spirit is a good thing.  God gave it to us for a purpose.  It is to get us to turn to him.  I cannot provide enough emphasis on this.  He is the only answer, and more food will never satisfy our soul.  Turn to God to meet your spiritual hunger.  Spend some time in His word or just talking to him about whatever is bothering you.  Journal it, writing a scripture prayer or other prayer.  It helps clear your mind. He will not fail to meet your need.  Psalm 107:9, "For he satisfieth the longing soul, and filleth the hungry soul with goodness."

1. What signals does your body give you that it is a genuine physical hunger versus emotional hunger?
2. What outside sources trigger a <u>false</u> hunger in you?
3. Which of the outside sources can you remove from your life?  How will you do this?
4. Is there anything else you can do to get away from the things that trigger a false hunger?  I.e., Advertisements, foods others are eating in your presence, photos on social media.
5. What can you do to renew your mind when a false hunger surfaces in your day?

# CHAPTER 17 - REJOICE IN SUFFERING

Romans 5:3-5 "And not only so, but we glory in tribulations also: knowing that tribulation worketh patience; And patience, experience; and experience, hope: And hope maketh not ashamed; because the love of God is shed abroad in our hearts by the Holy Ghost which is given unto us."

In other versions, the word "tribulations" translates as suffering.  I know the Apostle Paul wrote this, and his suffering or tribulations were not the same as ours.  His were fiercer and brought on more by other people, and circumstances than ours will ever be in this battle with the desire to eat more than we need.  That aside, the principle is the same.  The suffering still brings these results if we will glory, or rejoice, in the suffering.

When a person is trying to break through the desires of the body, the lusts of the flesh, it is not easy.  It is a battle in the mind and is a spiritual battle.  This battle often happens after a series of several weeks and successes with weight loss.  There is a battle that occurs after coming to the end of a "diet" and reaching a goal weight.

I have experienced this over and over in my life.  Many times, the week is going so well, I have stayed in boundaries, and I am sure my body is getting closer to the size and health God meant it to have.  I am feeling victorious.  Then a big temptation comes along.  There is an opportunity to eat something out of boundaries.

To go out of boundaries with my food is not something my spirit is wanting to do.  Like Jesus warned his disciples in Matthew 26:41, "Watch and pray, that ye enter not into temptation: the spirit indeed is willing, but the flesh is weak."

If you do fail, do not give up.  Confess it to God, and maybe confess to your accountability partners as well.  Receive God's forgiveness and go on.  For me, it is helpful to use the tool Barb Raveling has made, the "*I Deserve A Donut*" book or app.  It helps me think about what is causing the problem.  It also helps me understand how I can do better next time.

Hebrews 12:11 "Now no chastening for the present seemeth to be joyous, but grievous: nevertheless afterward it yieldeth the peaceable fruit of righteousness unto them which are exercised thereby."

There is purpose in suffering.  When you have won the battle, you will be stronger for the next fight. Strengthen your spiritual muscles.

The other half of this equation is to weaken the flesh while strengthening the spirit. Fasting is an excellent way to do this.  When we fast, the Spirit of God in us will begin to grow stronger, and the flesh becomes weaker.  If you cannot do a full fast, even a partial fast is helpful.   In the New Testament, Jesus gives an example of how fasting provides strength.  (Mark 9:29) In Acts, we see Cornelius receiving a message from God after fasting. (Acts 10:30) There are many more examples also.  If you have never fasted, give it a try.  It does not have to be a long fast. Start with even a short fast like 12 hours.  Or try fasting from a favorite food.  Pray about it and do what you feel God wants you to do.  It works.

I Corinthians 10:12 "There hath no temptation taken you but such as is common to man: but God is faithful, who will not suffer you to be tempted above that ye are able; but will with the temptation also make a way to escape, that ye may be able to bear it."

We can have success.  God will not give us a temptation or a challenge that we cannot successfully overcome. God knows what we can do.  Every time we pass a test, we have more strength.  We have more faith that we can do it again.  It is like practice.  The more you practice saying no to temptation, the easier it becomes. You will develop a new habit.

As a practical tip, I will share something I learned from one of the ladies in a weight loss group to which I belonged.   When a portion of food was out of her boundaries, she would say, "That is not my food."  This saying became a new habit for her.  I have used this a lot also.  If it is out of my boundaries, it is not my food.  If it is not my food, it is easier to say, "No, thank you" to it.

Developing new habits will increase your strength to overcome temptation.

The way of escape God gives us has to be put into use.  I will provide you with an example.  I have the temptation to eat something, a desert probably, that I know is more than what is allowed in my boundaries.  As I am bringing the bite to my mouth, I drop it on the floor.  Her is my perfect opportunity to say, "No, I will not eat that.  It has been on the floor."  Instead, my fleshly desire raises, and I say, "I want that even though I know, I should not have it."  I pick it up, wipe it off as best I can, and eat it.  That is a foolish decision.  I thank God that other times my better sense kicks in, and I say, "Oh, thank you, Jesus.  I know I should not eat that anyway."  I pick it up and throw it out.

Journal Questions:

1. Journal about a time you had a battle after you have had success?
2. What lessons can you learn from facing a challenge after losing weight?
3. What are the blessings you receive when you have faced a challenge and not fallen to temptation?
4. What will you do to strengthen your spiritual muscles?
5. Have you ever fasted?  Will you commit to a fast right now?  If so, what type of fast will you do and how long will it last?

6. Have you ever been successful in overcoming temptation with eating? If so, journal about your success.

7. Have you failed in overcoming temptation? If so, what can you learn and change for the next time?

8. Use one of the verses in this chapter in a renewing of the mind exercise. Some suggestions, write it on a card to remind yourself, write it into a prayer or personal application, memorize it and meditate on it.

9. Find a way that God relates to you in this scripture and thank him for being your protector in temptation.

# CHAPTER 18 - MY GOAL

Over the years, my "goal weight" changed. Change is normal. When I was younger, my goal was to get back to the size I was in High School. As I became a mother in my twenties, I realized it was not a reality. Ultimately, I have decided my goal is to be as healthy as it is reasonable for me. All of us have genetic predispositions for disease, and we can only do the best we can with what God has given us.

One of the things I added to my life was physical exercise. When I was at my heaviest weight, the best I could do was walk. I began very slowly. I couldn't go near as fast as I wanted to. I had done some running and speed walking before and enjoyed it, but in the beginning, it was not a possibility. Fortunately, I was in good enough health to begin a run program eventually.

God knows what our limits are. He does not expect more from us than we can do. As it is with our food boundaries, each of us will have different limitations for bodily exercise. Some people will just go walking. Some will only do housework.  For some persons, their job is physically taxing, and that is enough for them.

For those with a history of heart problems, there is a need for more.  Any exercise program should not begin without the approval of your primary physician.  Doing some type of aerobic exercise, which may be as simple as a very brisk walk, could be where you start.  Everyone's level of exertion will be different.

An easy tip I heard is to see how fast you can go and still speak without being out of breath.  If you can sing, then you could probably go more quickly.  Do, but don't over-do.

I will say again that your primary physician should approve any exercise.  As long as you are doing enough to stay healthy, it is enough.  We do not need to try out for the Olympics.

I have been able to lower my blood pressure and get off of blood pressure pills.  That has been a significant goal for me.  I was also able to decrease the dosage of my cholesterol medication, but cannot seem to get it low enough to get off it completely.  Be sure to consult with your primary healthcare provider before making any changes in your medications.

It is possible to be what the world would consider overweight, but also be very healthy.  This fact shows the importance of getting a physical check-up and becoming aware of any physical problems you may have.

Each person will be different.  For those of us with more serious family or personal health histories, it is essential to watch what we eat and to watch our weight.

My husband has been very healthy despite being overweight.  Even when he was more overweight than I was, his blood pressure was normal, and his cholesterol was in normal limits.  Those were not his lot.  He is blessed.

By increasing his physical activity and just cutting back a little on what he ate improved the few health problems he had.  His sugar level went back to normal from having been in the "Pre-diabetic" stage.

Journal questions:

1.  Is your goal a number on the scale, a health goal, or both?

2.  Do you think your goals are reasonable?

3.  When was the last time you had a physical exam?

4.  When is your next physical exam scheduled?

5.  Today, let's use the verse in, 1Corinthians 6:19 and 20 "What? know ye not that your body is the temple of the Holy Ghost which is in you, which ye have of God, and ye are not your own? For ye are bought with a price: therefore glorify God in your body, and in your spirit, which are God's."  for your

mind renewal.  Which method will you choose to use?

# CHAPTER 19 – WHERE DID MY SELF CONTROL GO?

There have been times when I felt I had surrendered everything to God and was no longer in captivity to the call of my flesh for more food than I needed. I would tell other people about it. I even testified in church, "God has blessed me. I am thankful. I no longer feel the pull to eat more than I need."

Then in a few months, I was out of control again. It is so embarrassing to regain the weight and let people see you overeating when you have told them you would never return there. It is especially awkward when you say to them, "God freed me from it."

What happened? Did God go back on his promise? Had God ever freed me? Or had I just been controlling it myself? I know the spirit of God in me is stronger than my flesh. The question is, what had I been strengthening? Had I been building God up in my soul? Or had I been leading my flesh into tempting situations? Had I been feeding the lusts of the flesh and letting those appetites revive?

We know the Bible tells us he will never leave us or forsake us. Hebrews 13:5b, "for he hath said, I will never leave thee, nor forsake thee."  I also know my flesh is not dead.  I am convicted by Paul's admission in I Corinthians 9:27 "But I keep under my body, and bring it into subjection: lest that by any means, when I have preached to others, I myself should be a castaway."  Even though I strive for perfection, I cannot give up.  It is a continual battle.  I thank God for the grace he gives.  1 John 1:9 says, "If we confess our sins, he is faithful and just to forgive us our sins, and to cleanse us from all unrighteousness."  John wrote the book of First John to Christians.  So, I know we are not the only ones who continue to need to go back and ask forgiveness again.

I am also encouraged by Paul in II Corinthians 12:7-10. He says, "And lest I should be exalted above measure through the abundance of the revelations, there was given to me a thorn in the flesh, the messenger of Satan to buffet me, lest I should be exalted above measure.  For this thing I besought the Lord thrice, that it might depart from me.  And he said unto me, My grace is sufficient for thee: for my strength is made perfect in weakness. Most gladly therefore will I rather glory in my infirmities, that the power of Christ may rest upon me. Therefore I take pleasure in infirmities, in reproaches, in necessities, in persecutions, in distresses for Christ's sake: for when I am weak, then am I strong."

I had to accept that this was the "thorn in the flesh" I had. I would just have to find a way to work with it for the rest of my life.  Because of this, I have accepted that I cannot forget this weakness of my flesh.  It is not as big a fight as it used to be, and for this, I am thankful, but I cannot pretend it is not there.  It helps me always to have some kind of devotional or study I am doing regarding this battle.   It also helps if I continually keep myself accountable to either a person or a small group.  When I let either of these practices go, I get a little too careless with my boundaries, and my health suffers.

Not giving up on this ongoing challenge helps grow us as Christians.  It works on our character.

Journaling questions:

1. How do you handle the embarrassment of going back to being overweight when you had been "successful?"
2. What triggers cause you to start overeating again?
3. I've given several verses in this chapter that you could use to apply to your life.  Which will you choose to use?
4. Consider memorizing and meditating on the scripture you choose.  Or write it on a card and keep it where you can see it often.  What will you do?

# CHAPTER 20 - WHY HAVE I NOT YET OVERCOME?

We have probably all been here.  We are still in bondage to the desire for too much food, but we want to be free. Whether or not we have falsely thought we were free or not, we desire to be free.

Does God do miracles?  I have seen too many set free from their bondage to drugs and alcohol, not to think it doesn't happen.  Does God always give this miracle to everyone that asks?

I used to teach a class in our church for those in bondage to drugs and alcohol.  We explained that it was possible, by the power of God, to be set free.  As I said, I saw those that were set free.  On the other hand, I saw some very sincere hearts, people who had a real love for God, who were not set free.  The desire for alcohol did not go away. These persons had to set strict boundaries for themselves. By God's help and the help of community or an accountability support person, they have stayed away from the alcohol.  Physiologically, food does not have the same physically addictive properties that drugs and alcohol do.  But there is no doubt it can have the same mentally addictive pull.  It can also cause a strong pull for the sensation you receive for specific properties of the food.  For many, it is the sugar; for others, it is the spice, and for some, it is a particular desire for the texture.

The decision to take this lust of the flesh captive and "put it to tribute" is the answer.  The boundaries given by God, have to be firm, no more bargaining or the fleshly desires will gain strength.   It can be hard to get free of the temptation to bargain our way into breaking our boundaries.  Use support.  It is necessary to stay in tune with God for help to continue in this decision.  It means there has to be a daily discipline of feeding your spirit. It is the only way to keep the Spirit of God stronger in your life than the lust of the flesh.  Use the scriptures you are learning to focus your mind on what God wants you to be doing.  Use these scriptures to renew the thinking in your mind.

There are many ways to feed the truth into your mind. Keep it up.  It does get easier to overcome temptation. The battle doesn't always go away completely, just like Paul's thorn in the flesh did not go away.  But it becomes easier to keep the flesh in subjection.  This problem that you have, with God's help, can be brought into subjection, it will lose strength.  The battle becomes shorter.

I want to encourage you.  Over time you will find your weight and health stabilize.  You will be able to stay in boundaries more often than not.  We must know, though, that we cannot become complacent. Remember what the apostle Peter says in I Peter 5:8-9 "Be sober, be vigilant; because your adversary the devil, as a roaring lion, walketh about, seeking whom he may devour: Whom resist stedfast in the faith, knowing that the same afflictions are accomplished in your brethren that are in the world."

Stay vigilant.  The devil isn't dead yet, and the flesh isn't either.  Some day the battle will be over, and we will rejoice in Heaven.  Until then, we continue.  To learn to think what God wants us to think, and to do what he wants us to do.

Journaling questions:

1.  Which of the mind renewal tools, or verses you have been using is helping your spirit gain strength and your fleshly desires lose power?
2.  Have you made your food boundaries firm and non-negotiable?  Write them down and post them somewhere for you to see daily. It doesn't mean you will never mess up unintentionally; it means you will not plan a mess up.
3.  What are you doing to get your mind into thinking the truth?
4.  Are you willing to commit to daily accountability? If you do not have an accountability partner or group, or both, it is time to find one.

5. If God has set you free from the lust for too much food, let others know.  Share the good news.  It is not impossible.

# PRACTICAL HELP AND TIPS

If you have a challenge with overeating good food, I will share a tip that has helped me.   Use a smaller plate. Those of us who like to finish what is on our plate find this very useful.  When we have a large plate, the appropriate sized serving looks so small. Then tell yourself, "No second helpings."

Here are some suggestions if you are eating too fast, and it seems the meal goes by at lightning speed.

A)  Use smaller utensils and take smaller bites.

B) Put your fork or spoon in your less dominant hand.  If you are right-handed, have you ever tried eating your soup with your spoon in your left hand?  It can get interesting.

C) Set your eating utensils down between each bite.

D) Take a sip of water between each bite.

If seeing food sets you off, walk away when a commercial for food comes on.  Or look away and check your text messages or posts on Facebook, anything to get your eyes off the tempting images.

Quit picking up magazines with diets and recipes in them. If there are things you want to read in a magazine, make yourself flip past the tempting photos quickly.

Unsubscribe to as many "food" oriented email lists as you can.  It is a matter of, "If your right hand offends you cut it off." If watching the cooking channel is tempting you, don't turn it on!!! If magazine pictures make you want to bake whatever it is, burn them!  Or recycle them.  You know what I mean.

When you walk in a restaurant, walk right past the dessert case and don't glance at it. Don't even order dessert unless you have planned for it.
Something else that has helped me a lot is to consider if I am hungry or thirsty.  These sensations can sometimes get confused in our bodies.  If I take a good drink of water and still feel the feeling, I know it is hunger.  I am surprised by the many times that the sensation is gone, and it was only thirst.

# FOR THE CURIOUS

Nowhere in this narrative have I mentioned how much weight I lost over the years.  It was never a straight down line.  It was more like a roller coaster, depending on where on the journey I was.  When on a diet I went down when I stopped, I went up. When I began to apply what I had learned in the Bible consistently, I quit spiking.  I was not at my highest weight at that time.  My highest weight, to my recollection, was 182 pounds.  I am only five foot one, at that time I may have been taller as I have shrunk about three-fourths of an inch over the years.  At my lowest, I was 115 pounds.  I have leveled out, hovering around 120 to 122.  This range is where I am when I weigh daily, or when I just follow my boundaries and keep my mind thinking as God wants me to and don't have a scale for a month, or six months.

I wanted to include this testimony, so you knew it really does work for weight loss if that is your goal.  For those with anorexia, it will also work.  The change is in your relationship with food.

May God bless you all.

www.ingramcontent.com/pod-product-compliance
Lightning Source LLC
Chambersburg PA
CBHW031145250726

48655CB00002B/851